Physical Training Simplified

Physical Training Simplified

Edward B. Warman

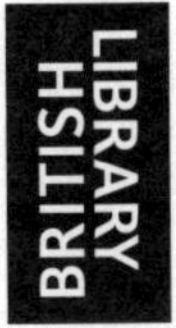

This edition published 2017 by
The British Library
96 Euston Road
London NW1 2DB

Originally published in 1911 by British Sports Publishing Co.

Cataloguing in Publication Data
A catalogue record for this book is available from the British Library

ISBN 978 0 7123 5683 1

Text designed and typeset by Tetragon, London
Printed in Malta by Gutenberg Press Ltd

Preface

PHYSICAL training is one of the great religions of the hour. Anything in connection with it should be of great concern. The exercises herewith given are so arranged as to meet the needs of the young, the middle-aged, and the aged of both sexes. Yes; the aged. One is never too old to reap some benefit. I recall, with pleasure, one pupil in Washington City who began at the age of 92. Another in Phœnix, Arizona, a good, old, motherly soul, who became so enthusiastic that, after our departure, she tried to kick a little ornament dangling from the centre of the chandelier. She said that she forgot, for the time being, that she was 87 years old.

This system is complete in itself, as it brings into healthful action every joint and every muscle of the body, and all of this *without the use of apparatus.*

Be it understood, however, that I am not opposed to heavy gymnastics, or to any form of apparatus that will give health, strength and confidence. To be so opposed would be inconsistent, from the fact that I take all of the muscular exercises with a pair of 5-lb. iron dumb-bells; but I have been a heavy-club performer for more than a quarter of a century, a catch-as-catch-can wrestler, and a heavy boxer; and, paradoxical as it may seem, a teacher of "Delsarte" for twenty years. (The Delsarte system, as far as exercise is concerned, is wholly æsthetic. It is not intended to make muscle, but to make *supple* the muscle already made; hence should not *supplant* but *supplement* the heavier work.) Nevertheless, I have realized the need of the publication of a system of exercises for those who cannot spare either money or time for the benefits of the gymnasium; for the thousands of men and women sedentarily employed; for the schools and colleges that have no apparatus or special room in which to exercise; hence this system, which it has been my pleasure to teach in every State and Territory, and in the Dominion of Canada. Therefore, it comes ripe from the school of experience.

Vigorously yours,

EDWARD B. WARMAN

Physical Training Simplified

"Multum in Parvo."

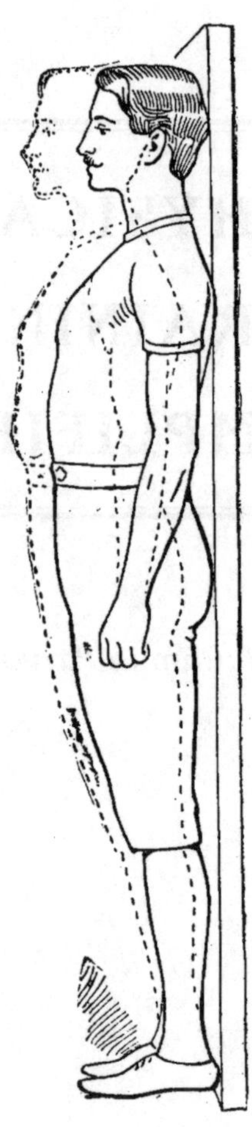

How to Stand

How to Stand

THE first essential is to obtain the *correct carriage of the body;* the next to *retain* it. This is important, not only as a matter of *grace*, but as a matter of *health.*

Carry your heart high is metaphorical; but to carry your stomach high is practical.

In order to obtain the correct carriage of the body one must learn *how to stand.* The weight of the body should be over the centre of the feet, about equally divided between the heel and the ball of the foot.

To obtain this position, stand against the wall, first touching the heels, then as much of the body as possible, drawing back the head to the wall, with the chin drawn slightly in. You will observe that the chest is expanded and in a firm position muscularly, thereby enabling you to retain the chest position independently of the breath.

This is only a means to an end; it is the first step towards securing correct position. Sway the entire body from the wall *without moving the feet,* moving no joint but the ankle joint. Thus it will be seen that the correct position consists of an active (firm) chest, abdomen drawn back, weight of the body off the heels, body erect.

If one is inclined to corpulency he is sure to sway back, sink the chest and protrude the abdomen—just the reverse of a correct position.

❦

How to Walk

The tendency is to allow the body to settle, thus making the legs do all the work. The chest should have the *appearance* of leading (the abdomen, never); the ball and the heel of the foot striking as nearly as possible simultaneously.

When having swayed from the wall, take a few steps, as if the first impulse came from the chest—onward and upward. You will observe a buoyancy and a lightness of step probably never before experienced. It will take but a short time until it will become a second nature, and you will feel uncomfortable in any other than a correct position.

How to Sit

Strange! Does not every one know how to sit? No; not for *health* and *strength.* If you doubt this, watch the children at school, the clerk at his desk, or anyone at the table during meals. The chair is too close to the desk or table, thus obliging the person to lean over until his spinal column is curved forward and his vital organs—heart, stomach and liver—are crowded. Indigestion, torpid liver, irregular heart action, headache, etc., etc., are sure to result.

Sit as far back in the chair as you can without allowing your back to touch the chair back; the spinal column as erect as when standing in a correct position. This will give you support for the base of the spinal column, and will allow your body to be as freely pivoted from the hips when sitting as it should be from the ankles when standing. Also, see to it that your chair is not too close to the desk or table.

How to Rest

How few persons know how to rest. Sitting is not always the equivalent of resting. If you want to rest thoroughly you must *let go*: let go mentally as well as physically; rest head, hand, foot, the entire being. If you rest easier and more satisfactorily by leaning back in the chair, then lean back and drive dull care to the winds.

If you become tired in reading or writing or studying; if the brain seems to lose its activity, its quickness of perception, its power of comprehension, there is nothing so good as some form of exercise—such as rising on the toes about forty or fifty times, slowly. This will draw the blood from the brain to supply the muscles; new blood will take its place, new tissue will be formed and the result will be increased brain activity with no ill results.

The best rest, however, for body and brain, especially the nerves, is the rest that should be taken by every one directly after the noon meal.

Sleeping at Will

This is the Spanish *siesta.* With the Spaniards and the Mexicans it is a necessity in their warm countries. It should be a necessity with every business man in our Northern countries. Instead of the Spaniard's two or more hours we need but fifteen minutes.

Any one should have so thorough discipline over self that he can go to sleep—or have sleep come to him—within two minutes. This is done by a process of:

Self Magnetizing

In order not to crowd the digestive organs, do not lie down after a hearty meal. Sit in an easy chair, one in which there is a rest for the head; or, any chair with a high enough back against which the head may rest. Tip the chair back, slightly. Place the feet on a chair as high or a trifle higher than the one upon which you are sitting. Cross the limbs at the ankles. Close the hands by putting finger between fingers interlacing, and the ends of the fleshy part of the thumbs together. Close the eyes. Breathe deeply. Think of nothing but the slow, measured breathing. You will be asleep in two minutes. Not the first time you try it, probably, but after a very few trials. Charge your mind with awakening in fifteen minutes. You can depend on it.

❦

Active Chest

An active chest is essential for correct breathing and perfect health. By an active chest I mean that the upper chest should be *raised* and *fixed,* independently of the breathing; fixed, as firm, as immovable as a wall, as far as involuntary breathing is concerned; fixed, even in voluntary breathing; fixed, in the most violent or vigorous physical or vocal exercises.

Place the hands upon the upper chest and allow the chest to become *passive;* to sink, as when that all-gone feeling sometimes comes to you. Then raise the chest *by the action of the muscles*, not by an inhalation.

You will soon discover how much muscular exercise (as well as thought) is required to *keep* your chest active without special effort and special thought at *all* times. This, *too,* must become a second nature. Do not go to the extreme and thereby invite attention to the disproportion and rigidity.

Breathing

Do not breathe through the lips. A dog breathes through the lips, but he holds a license from nature.

Correct breathing depends upon correct position. Stand erect, inclining the body slightly forward rather than backward. Do not bend the body, but incline it from the ankle; remove and avoid all rigidity; keep an active chest (raised and fixed); draw back the knees, hips and abdomen; throw the weight of the body toward and nearly over the ball of the foot; so much so that while still resting upon the heels the weight is so light thereon that one's fingers would not be hurt if placed underneath.

❦

Diaphragmatic Breathing

This includes the abdominal, costal and dorsal breathing; that is, front, side and back. Each of these it is necessary to treat separately.

In the following breathing exercises there should be no movement of the body except that caused by the action of the diaphragm and the waist muscles. Keep the upper chest *raised* and *fixed;* that is, put it there by a *muscular* movement (not by inhalation) and hold it there as if to receive a blow thereon. This position of the chest is of the utmost importance; hence, so constantly kept before the mind of the pupil, hoping thereby to get its importance *into* the mind and have it remain there.

❦

Abdominal Breathing

Inasmuch as the term is misleading, a word of explanation may prove helpful. Serious results have followed the practice of abdominal breathing, as it is generally understood. The *abdomen* does not breathe, the *chest* does not breathe, yet we have abdominal breathing and chest breathing.

Correct abdominal breathing is a healthful and invigorating exercise; for, in the contraction of the diaphragm, it presses upon the stomach and liver, which lie directly underneath. This movement upon the stomach is a promoter of good digestion. The term "abdominal breathing" derives its name from the forward movement of the abdomen during inspiration.

Stand in a correct position. (By this time correct position should be almost, if not entirely, a second nature.)

Place the tips of the fingers directly over the centre of the waist line. Take a deep inhalation through the nostrils very slowly. Keep the upper chest raised and fixed. There should be little or no movement below where the fingers are placed. It is not necessary, nor is it best, that the lower walls of

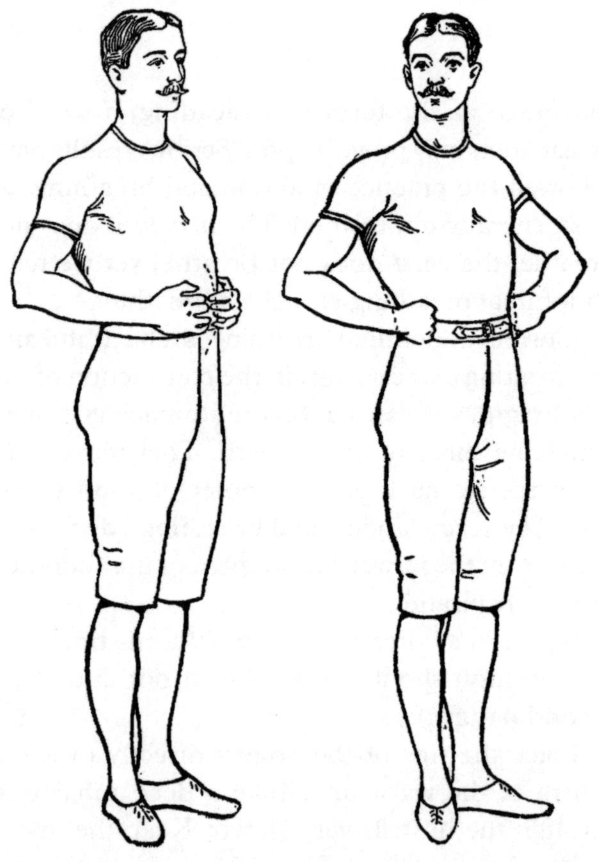

Abdominal Breathing *Intercostal Breathing*

the abdomen should move. The instant you begin to take the breath, you should feel a perceptible forward movement against your fingers. Inhale slowly, then check the diaphragm when the lungs are full, hold the diaphragm quiet a moment, then exhale slowly.

Abdominal Breathing—Place hands; inhale; check diaphragm; exhale slowly.

NOTE—Three times will suffice for *class* work; for *individual* work, each one must be guided by his own judgment.

❦

Costal Breathing

Stand in a correct position. Place the backs of the fingers against the lower ribs. Take a deep inhalation through the nostrils, very slowly. Keep the upper chest raised and fixed. The instant you begin to take the breath you should feel a perceptible sidewise movement against your fingers.

Costal Breathing—Place hands; inhale; check diaphragm; exhale slowly.

NOTE—Three times will suffice for *class* work; for *individual* work each one must be guided by his own judgment.

Dorsal Breathing

Stand in a correct position; chest active. Place the thumbs against each side of the base of the spinal column, keep them there by firm pressure, take a deep inhalation through the nostrils, very slowly. The instant you begin to take the breath you should feel a perceptible outward movement against the thumbs.

Dorsal Breathing—Place hands; inhale; check diaphragm; exhale slowly.

Note—Three times will suffice for *class* work; for *individual* work, each one must be guided by his own judgment.

Belt Breathing

The combination of the abdominal, intercostal and dorsal breathing constitutes what I term *Belt Breathing.*

Chest Expander—Place hands; inhale; forward—back; forward—back; exhale.

NOTE—For *class* work three times is sufficient; for *individual* work, each one must be his own guide.

❦

SHOULDER BRACE

Place the arms at side, as shown in the illustration. Extend the arms forward in a horizontal and parallel position, the muscles relaxed, hands open, palms downward.

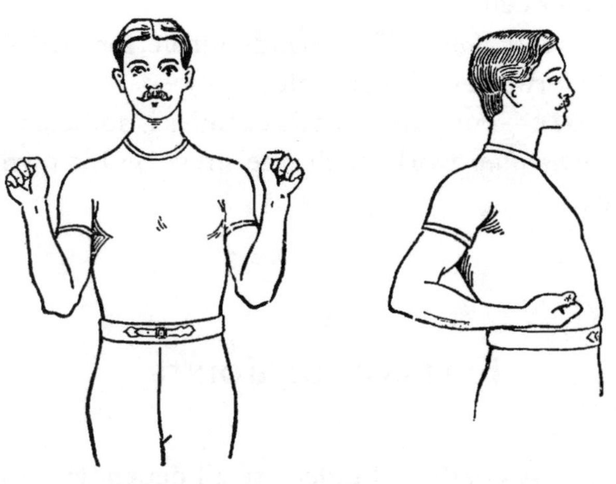

Chest Expander ***Shoulder Brace***

Slowly raise the hands, close them firmly. Draw the arms back slowly, the elbows leading. Keep the elbows up until they have passed back as far as possible. (During all this time the arms will be gradually closing.) Then slowly lower the elbows slightly, allowing the closed hands to turn, with fingers upward, but with hands still closed, the little fingers pressing against the ribs, *wrists unbent.*

After learning the movement, take a deep inhalation, and *hold* it from the time you place the arms in position until they return to position the second time. Make each *exhalation* as complete as possible, that the following *inhalation* may expand every air cell.

Shoulder Brace—Place hands; inhale; forward—back; forward—back; exhale.

NOTE—For *class* work three times is sufficient; for *individual* work, each one must be his own guide.

FREEDOM OF JOINTS

Health, strength and grace are all dependent, to a certain extent, upon the freedom of the joints.

These are simple, yet effective. If exercised every day, regularly and judiciously, stiffness of joints and rheumatism of the joints would be unknown.

❦

Fingers

Place the arms at the side. Raise the forearms in front until the hands are somewhat higher than the elbows. Keep the elbows against the side. Put sufficient force in the forearms and hands to differentiate and devitalize the fingers while thrusting the hands up and down continuously.

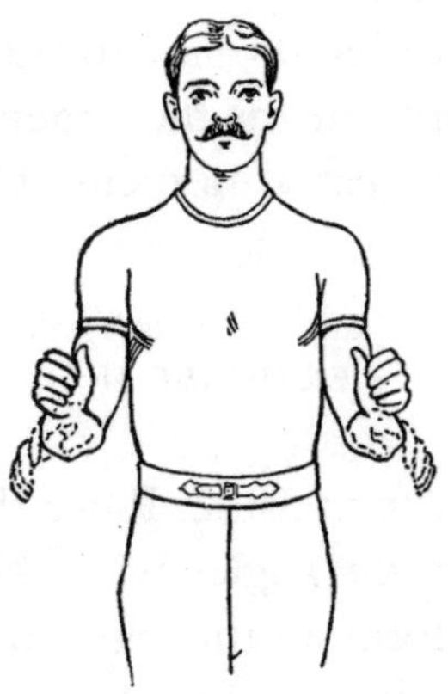

Fingers

Fingers—Place hands; thrust, rest; thrust, rest; thrust, rest.

NOTE—Continue the thrusting for a few seconds only, then rest a moment. Then again and again.

WRISTS

EXERCISE I

Place the arms at the side. Raise the forearms in front until at right angles with the upper arms. Put sufficient force in the forearms to move the hands from *side* to *side,* while keeping the elbows comparatively quiet.

Wrists—Place hands; side to side; rest.

NOTE—Continue the movement for a few seconds only, then rest a moment. Then again and again.

EXERCISE II

Place the arms at the side. Raise the forearms in front until at right angles with the upper arms. Put sufficient force in the forearms to move the hands *up* and *down,* while keeping the elbows comparatively quiet.

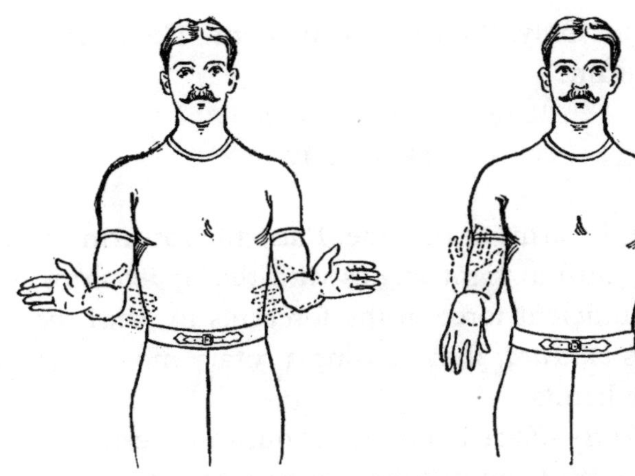

Wrists—Exercise I ***Wrists—Exercise II***

Wrists—Place hands; up and down; rest.

NOTE—Continue the movement for a few seconds only, then rest a moment. Then again and again.

EXERCISE III

Place the arms at the side. Raise the forearms in front until at right angles with the upper arms. Put sufficient force in the forearms to whirl the arms *inward*, thus causing a rotary movement of the hands.

Wrists—Place hands; whirl inward; rest.

NOTE—Continue the movement for a few

seconds only, then rest a moment. Then again and again.

EXERCISE IV

Place the arms at the side. Raise the forearms in front until at right angles with the upper arms. Put sufficient force in the forearms to whirl the hands *outward,* thus causing a rotary movement of the hands.

Wrists—Place hands; whirl outward; rest.

NOTE—Continue the movement for a few seconds only, then rest a moment. Then again and again.

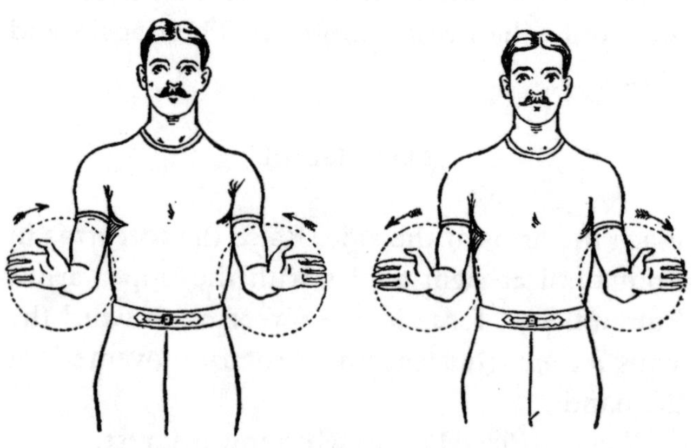

Wrists—Exercise III ***Wrists—Exercise IV***

❦

Elbows

EXERCISE I

Place the left hand to the side, the arm akimbo. Bend the body to the left, at the same time raising the *right* arm until the elbow is about even with the shoulder. Put sufficient force in the upper arm to swing the forearm and hand backward and forward. There should be no life, apparently, in the forearm.

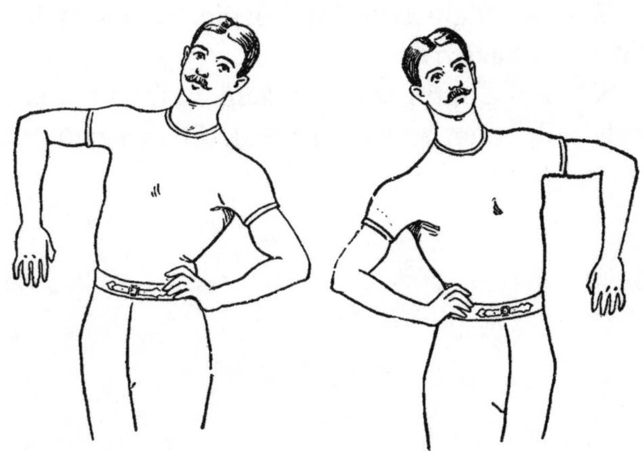

Elbows—Exercise I ***Elbows—Exercise II***

Elbows—Left arm akimbo; place right arm; forward and back; rest.

NOTE—Continue the movement for a few seconds only, then rest a moment. Then again and again.

EXERCISE II

Place the right hand to the side, the arm akimbo. Bend the body to the right, at the same time raising the *left* arm until the elbow is about even with the shoulder. Put sufficient force in the upper arm to swing the forearm and hand backward and forward. There should be no life, apparently, in the forearm.

Elbows—Right arm akimbo; place left arm; forward and back; rest.

NOTE—Continue the movement for a few seconds only, then rest a moment. Then again and again.

Shoulders

EXERCISE I

Allow both arms to hang apparently lifeless from the shoulders. Put sufficient force in the chest and shoulders to twist the body quickly to the left. This must be done by one impulse. Allow both arms to sway freely, but bring the body back to position. Do not repeat the impulse until the arms cease swaying.

Shoulders—Impulse to the left; rest.

Note—Repeat each impulse when the arms cease swaying.

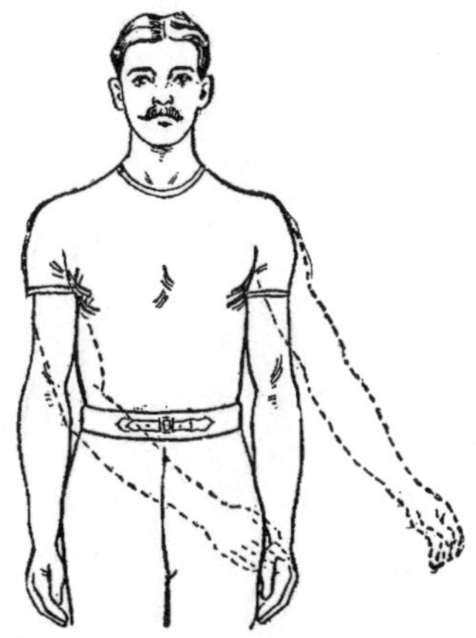

Shoulders—Exercise I

EXERCISE II

Allow both arms to hang apparently lifeless from the shoulders. Put sufficient force in the chest and shoulders to twist the body quickly to the right. This must be done by one impulse. Allow both arms to sway freely, but bring the body back to position. Do not repeat the impulse until the arms cease swaying.

Shoulders—Impulse to the right; rest.

NOTE—Repeat each impulse when the arms cease swaying.

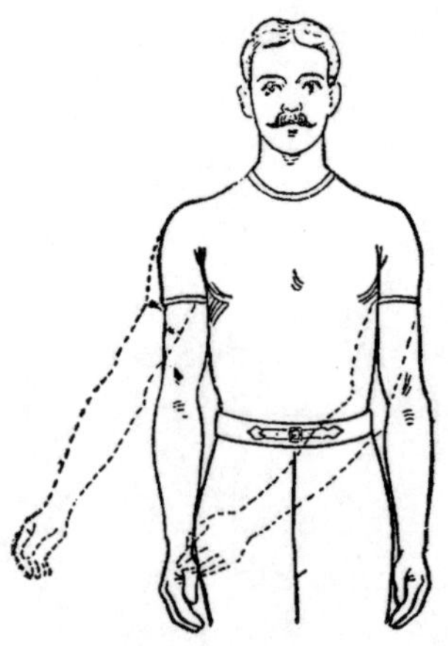

Shoulders—Exercise II

Neck

EXERCISE I

The benefits derived from the neck exercises are two-fold: first, the freedom of the joints; second, the developing and strengthening of the *muscles* of the neck, and, at the same time, *covering the scrawny neck* (especially the scare-crow bone) with good solid flesh. In order to accomplish this it is necessary to go beyond the devitalizing exercises usually given for this purpose by teachers of the Delsarte æsthetic exercises.

Slowly bow the head forward and downward as far as possible, stretching the neck muscles to the utmost without yielding the slightest at the waist muscles; that is, without swaying. Raise the head slowly, and as slowly bow it as far back and down as possible.

These exercises must not be done in a careless, listless manner, but with a *purpose* underneath. Avoid jerkiness.

Neck—Forward, raise; backward, raise.

NOTE—Three times each way will suffice for *class* work.

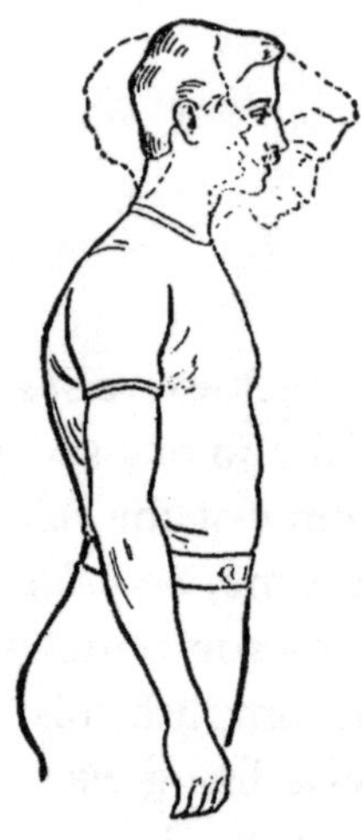

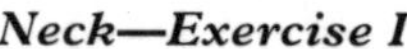

Neck—Exercise I

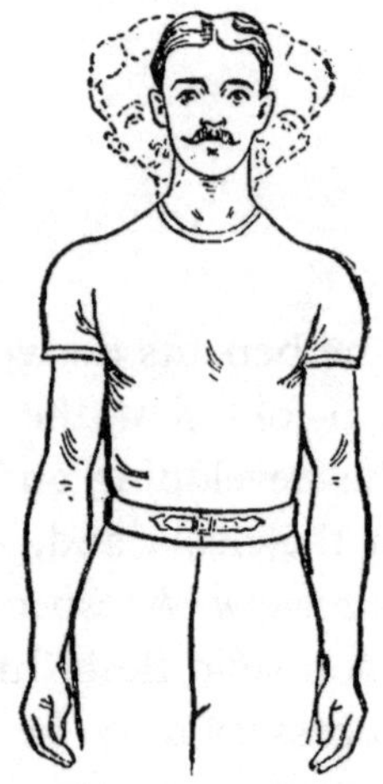

Neck—Exercise II

EXERCISE II

Slowly lower the head sidewise toward the left shoulder stretching the muscles to the utmost. Do not allow the body to sway or bend, nor the head to turn, nor the shoulder to rise. Raise the head slowly, and as slowly lower it sidewise toward the right shoulder. Do not allow the body to sway or bend, nor the head to turn, nor the shoulder to rise.

Neck—Left, raise; right, raise.

NOTE—Three times each way will suffice for *class* work.

EXERCISE III

Have the head perfectly poised, then slowly turn it to the *left* until, if possible, a perfect profile is formed. Keep the head erect and the body immovable. Then as slowly turn the head back to the front position, then to the *right* until, if possible, a perfect profile is formed. Keep the head perfectly poised.

The question may be asked concerning the rotary movement of the head. I have discarded it since using the *stretching* instead of the *devitalizing* exercises of the neck.

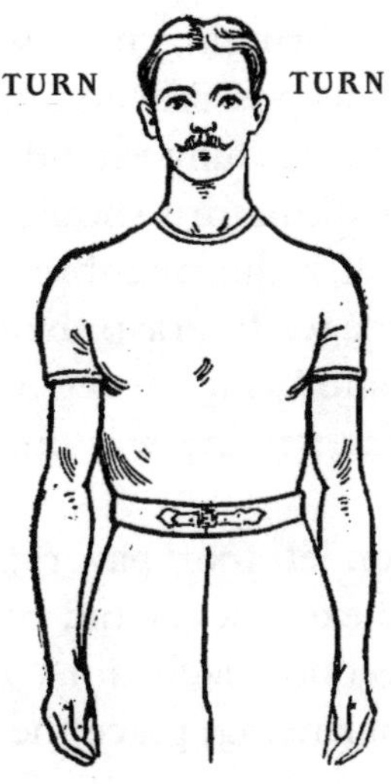

Neck—Exercise III

Neck—Left, turn, front; right, turn, front.

NOTE—Three times each way will suffice for *class* work.

HIPS

EXERCISE I

Stand erect, with the weight of the body on the left foot. *Paw* with the *right* foot by first drawing it far back, then bringing it forward by raising the knee as high as possible and pushing the foot forward until the leg is fully extended. The position of the leg at this juncture should be very much that of the leg of a thoroughbred trotter just as the foot seems eager to grasp the turf. Strike the ball of the foot and bring the leg back to position, and continue the pawing without halting at the starting point.

Hip—Settle on left foot; paw right; rest.

NOTE—This exercise should be continued for a number of seconds each time. If at first there is difficulty in balancing, place the left hand on a chair or desk.

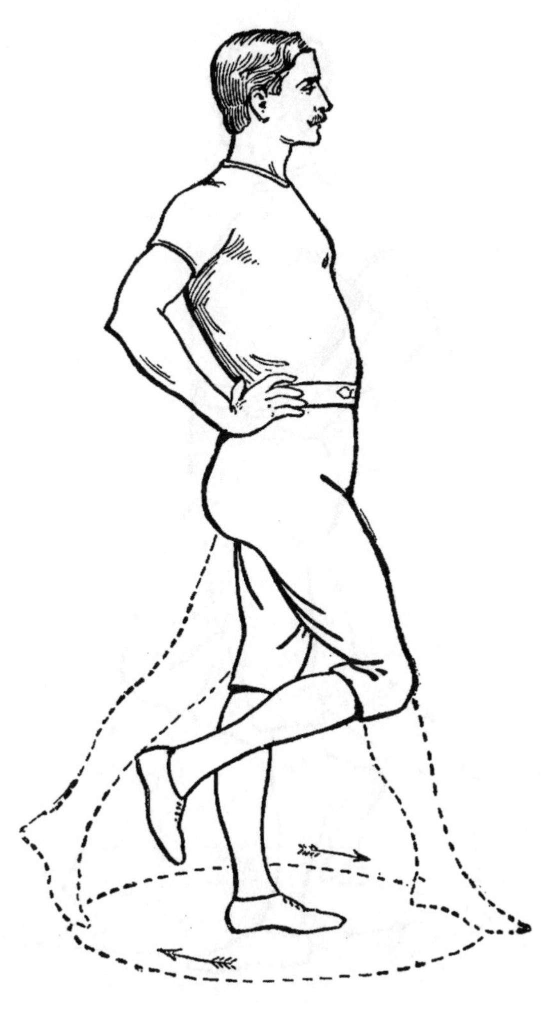

Hips—Exercise I

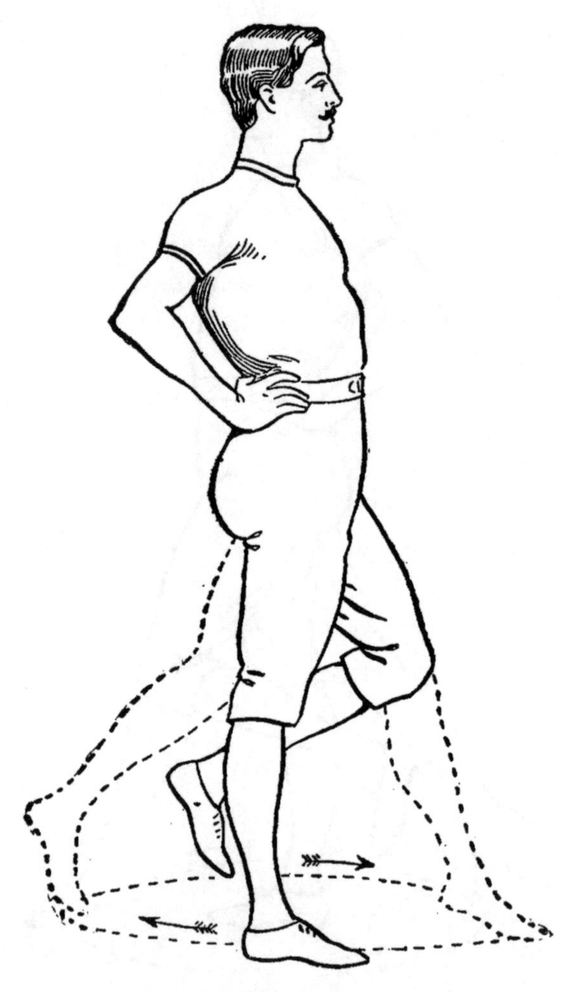

Hips—Exercise II

EXERCISE II

Stand erect, with the weight of the body on the right foot. *Paw* with the *left* foot by first drawing it far back, then bringing it forward by raising the knee as high as possible and pushing the foot forward until the leg is fully extended. Strike the ball of the foot and bring the leg back to position, and continue the pawing without halting at the starting point.

After practising vigorously for a short time with both legs, place the hands on the hips, walk a few steps and note the almost immediate benefit.

One can hardly realize that so little exercise can produce so good results.

Hip—Settle on right foot; paw left; rest.

NOTE—This exercise should be continued for a number of seconds each time. In *class* work, the teacher should use his or her discretion as to the number of times.

Knees

EXERCISE I

Stand erect, with the weight of the body on the left foot. Raise the *right* knee until the calf of the leg touches the thigh. Place the foot to the floor quickly but noiselessly.

Knee—Settle on left foot; right; up, down.

Note—Continue this exercise for a number of seconds. In *class* work, the teacher should use his or her discretion as to the number of times.

EXERCISE II

Stand erect, with the weight of the body on the right foot. Raise the *left* knee until the calf of the leg touches the thigh. Place the foot to the floor quickly but noiselessly.

Knee—Settle on right foot; left; up, down.

Note—Continue this exercise for a number of seconds. In *class* work, the teacher should use his or her discretion as to the number of times.

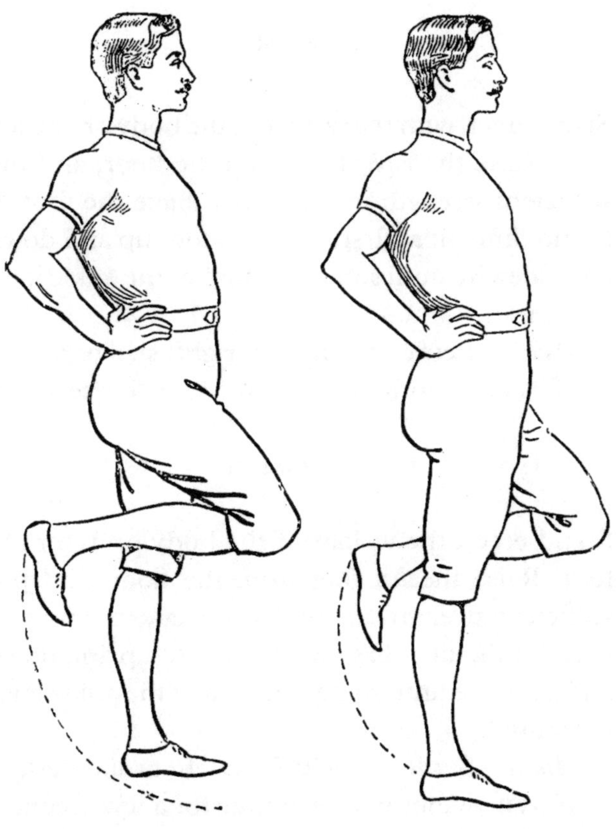

Knees—Exercise I *Knees—Exercise II*

Ankles

EXERCISE I

Stand erect, with the weight of the body on the left foot. Raise the *right* foot from the floor, and put sufficient strength in the leg to shake the foot. If found difficult at first, work the foot up and down and sidewise until some freedom of the ankle joint is secured.

Ankle—Settle on left foot; right; shake; rest.

NOTE—Continue each time for a few seconds.

EXERCISE II

Stand erect, the weight of the body on the right foot. Raise the *left* foot from the floor, and put sufficient strength in the leg to shake the foot. If found difficult at first, work the foot up and down and sidewise until some freedom of the ankle joint is secured.

Ankle—Settle on right foot; left; shake; rest.

NOTE—Continue each time for a few seconds.

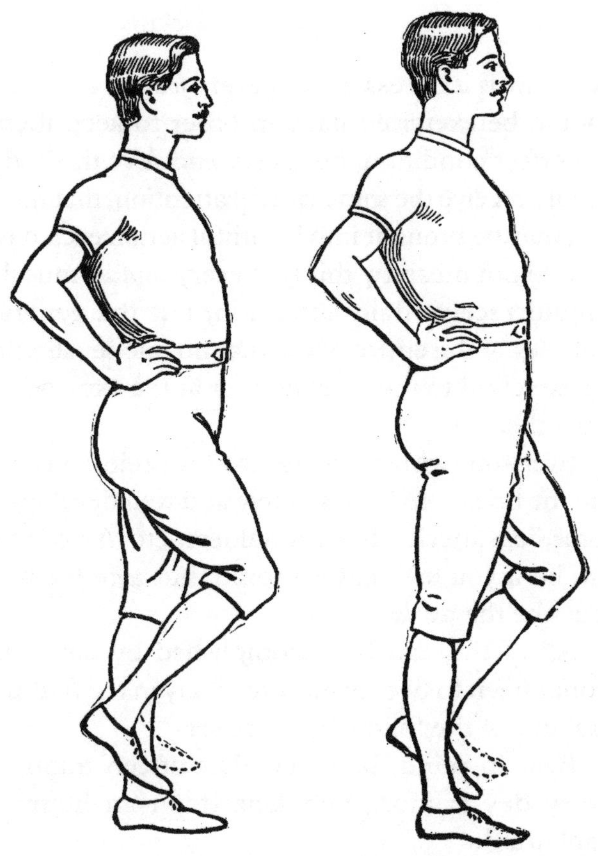

Ankles—Exercise I   *Ankles—Exercise II*

A Word About the Muscles

Not only is it necessary that every *joint* of the body should be exercised daily in order to keep them in perfect condition, but every *muscle* of the body should receive the same careful attention, that they, too, may be brought into healthful action each day.

I do not mean by this that every *minute* muscle should receive daily attention, but the general muscles of the entire body; that no one set should be exercised to the detriment or at the expense of any other set.

Every one wishes—if one has any pride concerning the body—to have shapely and well developed arms, legs, neck, chest, shoulders, etc. All of this *can* be if you *will* that it should, but *with* the will must be the *work*.

All of this can be accomplished by devoting from fifteen to twenty minutes a day in the faithful practice of the following exercises.

Bear in mind, however, that fifteen minutes every day is more beneficial than an hour at haphazard.

❦

Forearms

EXERCISE I

There are two special exercises for the development of the forearm muscles.

While the arms are pendent at the side, close the hands firmly and then open quickly and vigorously until the fingers are extended to the utmost. Continue the rapid and vigorous opening and closing of the hands with as little movement as possible of the arms.

Forearms—Hands shut; open (ten times each).

Note—For special individual work, not less than twenty-five to fifty times each.

EXERCISE II

Extend the arms full length at the side, horizontally. Close the hands firmly, palms down. Draw the hands as far *down* and *under* as you can, then raise them as *high* as possible. Both of these movements—up and down—should be done *without moving the arm, except at the wrist joint.*

N. B.—Although these movements *can* be given *without apparatus,* I think it better that the hands should grasp some light object; a dumb-bell not being objectionable. In place of the dumb-bell, however, I would especially recommend—for all of these exercises where dumb-bells can be used—the *Warman Grip Exerciser*, only 25 cents a pair, beautifully ebonited.

Forearms—Extend; down, up (ten times each).

NOTE—Stretch the muscles to the utmost, and by the time you have drawn the hands down and up ten times, you will feel the congestion of the blood in the forearm muscles. Not less than twenty-five times for special work.

❦

UPPER ARMS

EXERCISE I

There are two special exercises also for the *upper arms:* The first for the *biceps* and the *triceps;* the *lifting* and the *striking* muscles. These develop the arm front and back and give it a shapely and graceful appearance when viewed from the side.

Extend the arms full length at the side, horizontally, palms up. Close the hands, as if firmly grasping a dumb-bell. Bring the hands in vigorously

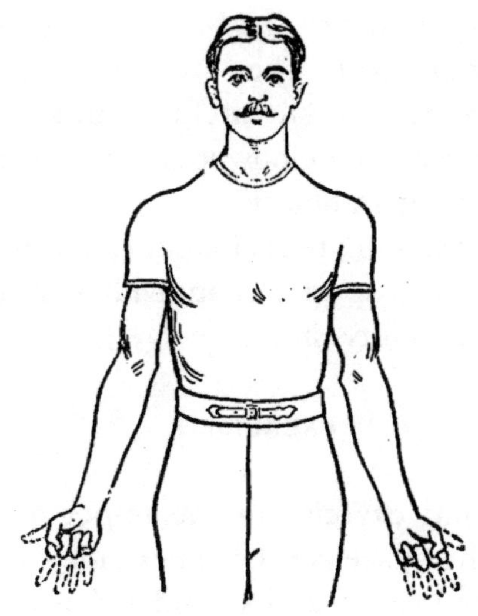

Forearms—Exercise I

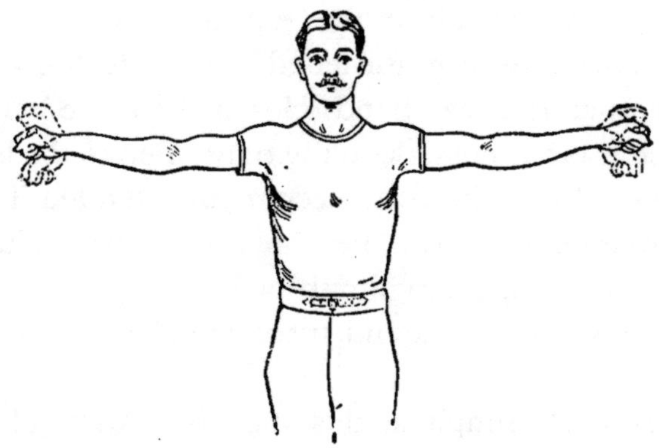

Forearms—Exercise II

toward the shoulders, *without lowering the elbows or bending the wrists.* Then strike them out to the starting point; at first, carefully, until you know the strength of your elbow joints, then vigorously, as if striking at an object.

Upper Arms—Extend; in, out (ten times each).

NOTE—For special or individual work, from twenty-five to fifty times.

EXERCISE II

This second exercise of the upper arms is to develop the space on the outer side of the arm between the elbow and shoulder that is so often lacking in otherwise well developed arms. This lack of development is especially noticeable when viewing the arm from the front or back.

Extend the arms full length at the side, horizontally, palms down, hands closed. Turn the hands over as far as possible to the right, then to the left. Do not lower the arms; keep them extended. This movement will affect the whole arm and shoulder. Grasp an imaginary dumb-bell.

Upper Arms—Extend; turn; right, left (ten times each).

NOTE—Simple as this appears, I know of no exercise more tiresome, if rightly done. For special or individual work, twenty times will suffice.

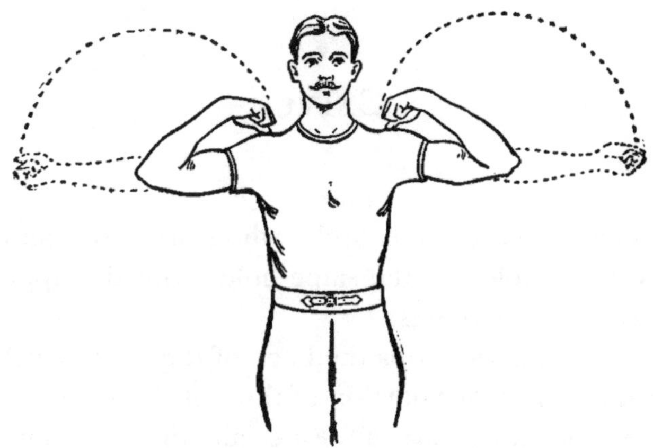

Upper Arms—Exercise I

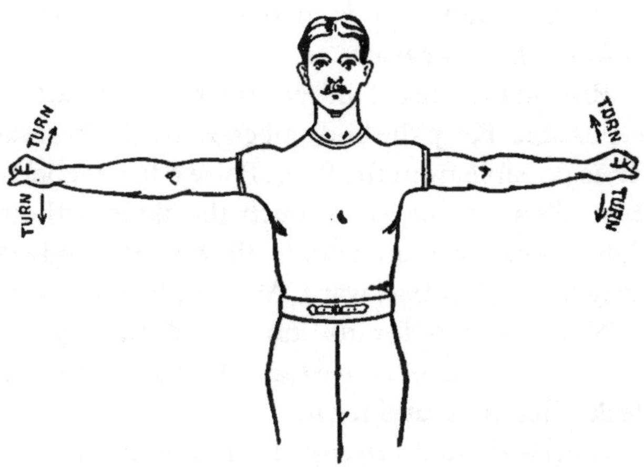

Upper Arms—Exercise II

Calves

What the forearm is to the whole arm, the calf is to the whole leg; the same holds with the upper arm and the thighs.

Walking develops the back of the calf; bicycle riding the outer portion of the calf. *This* exercise develops the *whole* calf, especially the *inner-upper* portion which, most of all, gives it the desired shapeliness.

When the calf of the limb is viewed from the side only, we cannot say it is shapely; not until viewed from the front or back.

Rise on the balls of the feet as far toward the toes as possible. Keep the body erect. Raise the heels as far as possible from the floor. Poise a few seconds, then allow the heels to touch the floor without sinking heavily upon them or allowing the body to sway forward or backward. Also, *walk* on the toes.

N. B.—A cure for insomnia, *a relief at any time to the overworked or weary brain.* Get up from your desk when tired and try it.

Calves—Rise slowly; up, down (ten times each).

Note—For special needs, from twenty-five to fifty times.

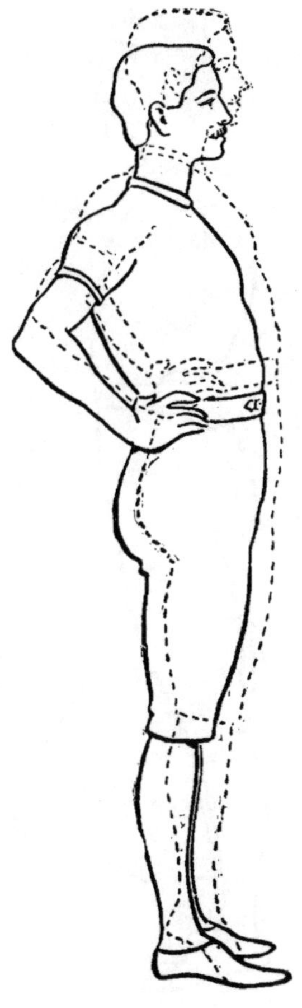

Calves

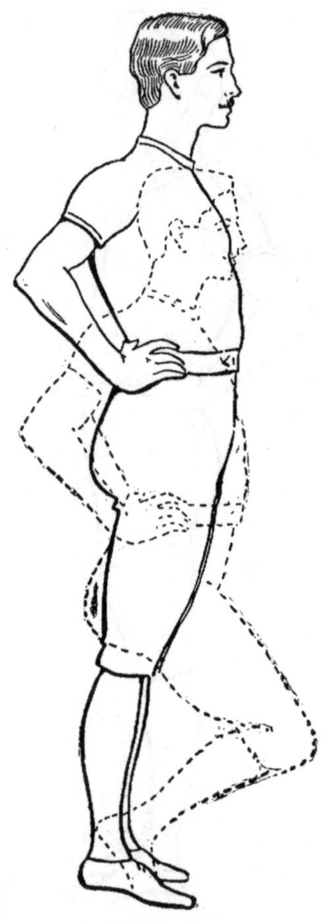

Thighs

❦

Thighs

The elasticity of one's step depends almost entirely upon the thigh muscles, and not, as is generally supposed, upon the calf muscles.

Stand erect. Settle the body quickly by bending the knees and lifting the heels from the floor, the entire weight of the body being upon the balls of the feet. Keep the upper portion of the body as erect as possible, even when sitting. Rise quickly.

After learning to keep your balance when in the sitting posture, jump about a number of times without rising to position.

There is no exercise to *compare* with this for stretching and developing the thigh muscles.

Thighs—Sit; rise (only five times each at first). Then jump while sitting.

Note—For special work, not less than twenty-five times.

Shoulders and Chest

EXERCISE I

There are four special exercises, three of which can be given with or without apparatus.

Stand erect, the arms pendent. Grasp an imaginary dumb-bell and turn the arms to the right until the palms of the hands are from the body, the back of the hands touching the limbs. Extend

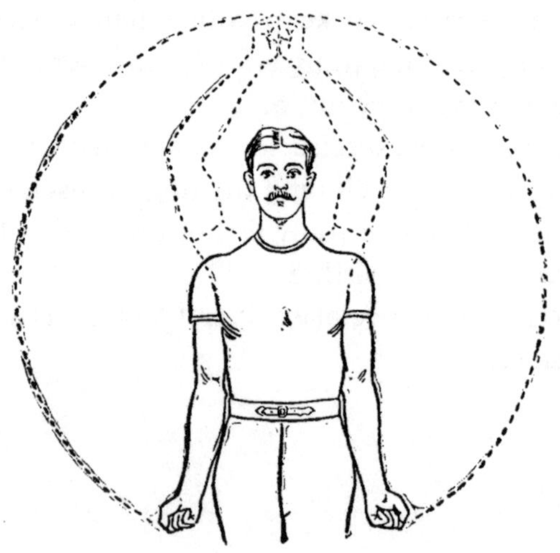

Shoulders and Chest—Exercise I

the arms outward and up until the closed hands touch above the head—as far above as possible. Bring the hands back to the sides of the body with the arms still extended.

Imagine you are lifting heavy dumb-bells, thus requiring the movement to be slow and as with effort. Lower them as if heavy and needing effort to meet the resistance.

Shoulders and Chest—Arms side; turn; up; down (ten times each).

NOTE—For special work, not less than twenty times.

EXERCISE II

Stand erect, arms pendent. Bring the hands up straight at the *side,* arms fully extended, until the hands and arms are about on a level with the shoulders. Grasp an imaginary dumb-bell in each hand, the dumb-bell being held upright. Bring the hands forward directly in front, arms fully extended; touch the closed hands, and then slowly return them to position and as far back as possible *without lowering the hands beneath the level of the shoulders*. Allow the body to sway from the ankle joints, but not to bend from the waist. Do not allow a forward movement of the head; that is, in advance of the body.

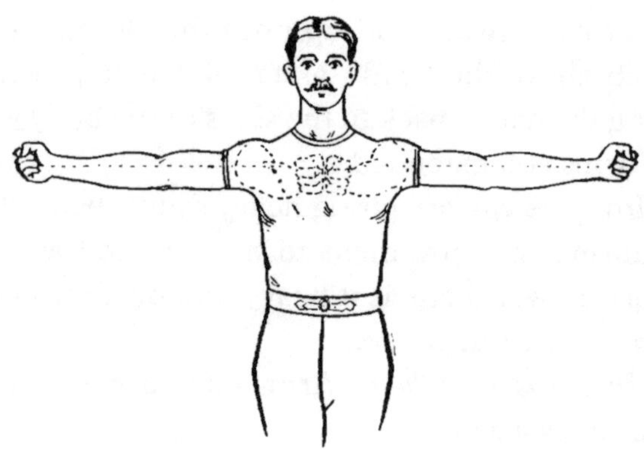

Shoulders and Chest—Exercise II

Shoulders and Chest—Arms side; up; front; back (ten times each).

NOTE—For special work, not less than twenty times.

EXERCISE III

Extend the right arm forward. Grasp an imaginary dumb-bell or Indian club and sweep it down toward the floor close to the side of the body. Continue the movement back and up until it has made a complete circle *without bending the arm at the elbow joint.*

Reverse the movement—after sweeping it forward from five to ten times. Do not allow the arm to bend; better that the entire body should twist from the ankles.

The same exercise (forward and reverse) should be taken with the *left* hand. The hand should make a perfect circle, following an imaginary line on the wall in front, the line continuing on the floor, up the wall behind you, straight across the ceiling to the line forming the starting point.

Shoulders and Chest—Right arm, front; sweep (ten); reverse (ten). Left arm, front; sweep (ten); reverse (ten).

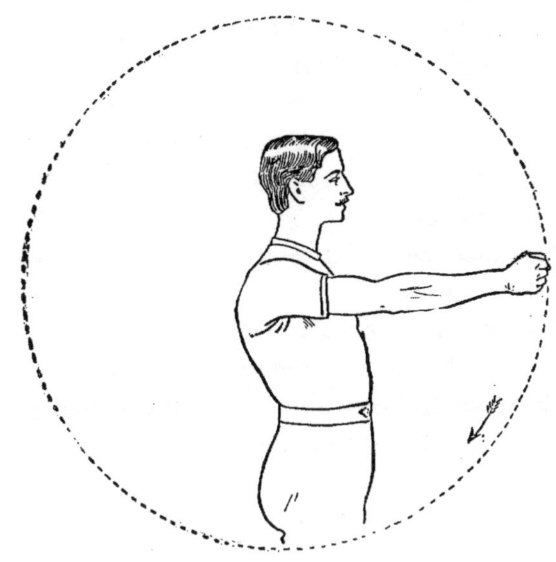

Shoulders and Chest—Exercise III

NOTE—For special work, not less than twenty times *each* way with *each arm.*

EXERCISE IV

Stand erect between two desks or chairs, or in front of a chair with high arms. Bend forward and place the hands upon the arms of the chair. Grasp them firmly. Step back until only the toes touch the floor. Hold up the head so that the body is straight from head to foot. Drop the body slowly between the desks or chairs or chair arms, dropping the body as low as the arms will admit.

To return: Straighten the arms slowly, raising the weight of the body resting upon them. *Do not bend the body when straightening the arms.*

This exercise is excellent also for the tricep (the striking muscle).

Shoulders and Chest—Chair; hands; feet; down; up (three times).

NOTE—This is a very difficult exercise if done correctly; that is, *not bending the body.* For class work, from three to five times; individual work, from ten to fifteen times.

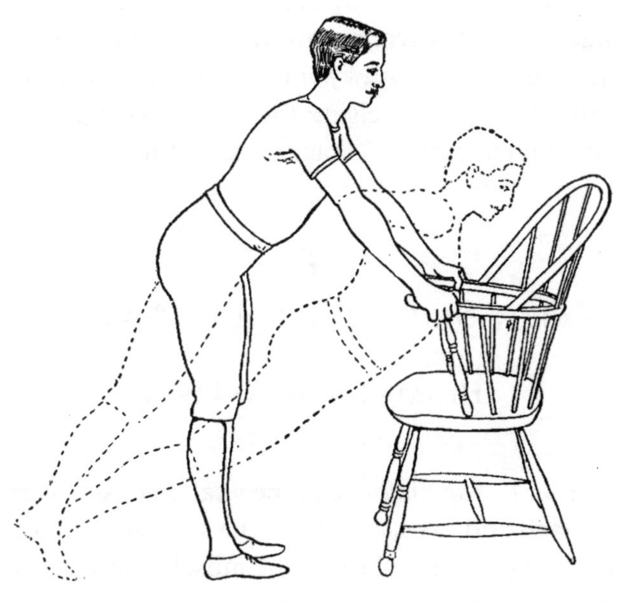

Shoulders And Chest—Exercise IV

Neck

Special exercises for the neck muscles are given on page 33. In the exercises given for the freedom and suppleness of the *neck joint*, they have been given with a view of exercising the *muscles* at the same time; hence, not necessary to repeat here.

Waist, Sides, Back and Abdomen

Heart—Stomach—Liver

In order to *habitually* carry the vital organs—heart, stomach and liver, especially the stomach—in the correct position for health, the muscles *surrounding* these organs should receive special attention.

There are no better exercises to secure the needed result than the three which I designate as Bowing, Bending, Twisting.

All of these have been taught and practised for years, but not with a view to any *special purpose;* hence, have not produced the needed results. So valuable are these three exercises in the *ob*taining and retaining of health that they should *precede* and *succeed* all others; in fact, they are of so great importance they could *supersede* all others. They care for that portion of the body almost wholly neglected by the average gymnast—the *health* of the *vital centres.*

If the demand of the muscles that waste exceeds the vital supply, no matter how strong the muscles are, impairment of health is inevitable.

Before beginning these exercises, a word, by way of encouragement, to show the benefits to be derived therefrom.

Special Benefits

First A friendly relationship between the heart, stomach and liver.

Second Retaining one's youthful spirits while growing old gracefully.

Third Retaining one's suppleness, even to and past three score and ten.

Fourth Preventing the bent and rigid form so common to old age.

Fifth Preventing and curing *obesity;* burning out the adipose tissue, and giving healthy, solid flesh instead.

Sixth Adding years to one's life and life to one's years.

Bowing

Stand erect. Place the hands on the hips. Raise the chest muscularly. Draw the hips and abdomen back as you bend the body forward slowly and as low as possible—so low that you feel a strong tension of the muscles on the back part of the legs. Keep the head up sufficiently to prevent an excess of blood in the head. *Do not bend the knees.*

Rise slowly to position and bend the body backward, *bending the knees* in order to prevent an undue strain that might possibly cause rupture. Keep your balance, even though you raise the heels from the floor.

After learning the position of the body—a few times' practice will suffice—instead of keeping the hands on the hips, raise them high above the head, as the chest and abdomen are lifted thereby. Swing the extended arms backward over the head, swaying the body as you go back, bend the knees slightly, and then swing forward, weight solid upon both feet, *knees unbent;* try to touch the floor with the fingers. Note how far your fingers are from the floor when you begin, and you will be encouraged when, by and by, you can touch the fingers, then the knuckles when the hands are closed, and finally the palm of the hands. Remember that the knees should not be bent when bending *forward.*

HOW OFTEN?

If you are unaccustomed to the exercise be satisfied with *five* times each way every day the first week; then *increase* five times each additional week until you reach fifty times each way every day.

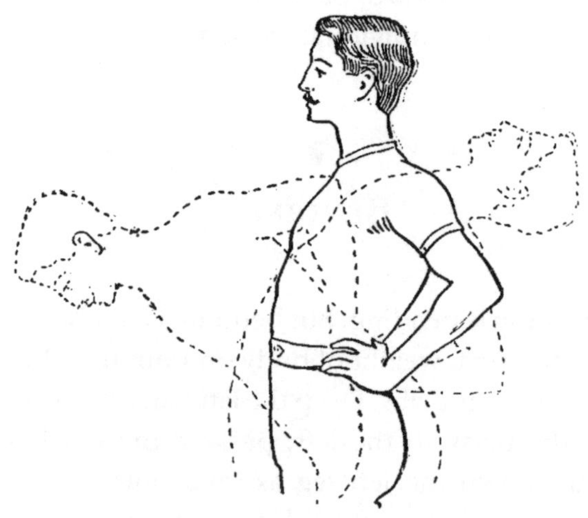

Bowing—Waist Muscles

For *many years* I have not missed taking my fifty bows every morning as soon after arising as convenient, no matter what the conditions or surroundings; sometimes in a sleeper; sometimes when getting ready to take a train at one, two or three o'clock in the morning; sometimes on an ocean steamer, when I am seriously meditating about casting my bread upon the waters; sometimes in a "spare room" (kept for ministers), the mercury dropping to 16 below zero; but always I bow, and always *fifty*.

Bowing—Forward, back (five times).

NOTE—For individual work, fifty times.

BENDING

Yes; bowing is bending, but bending is not bowing.

Stand erect, weight of body on both feet. Place the hands on the ribs. Drop the left hand and slowly bend the body to the left, passing the left hand straight down the left leg as far below the knee as possible. This must be done *without moving the right foot from the floor.*

Rise slowly. When back to position place the *left* hand on the ribs, drop the *right* hand, passing it straight down the right leg as far below the knee as possible. This must be done *without lifting the left foot from the floor.* Keep both feet firmly upon the floor during the bending to right and left.

Bending—Right, left (five times).

NOTE—Inasmuch as the *bowing* exercises all the waist muscles, ten times each way is sufficient for special work.

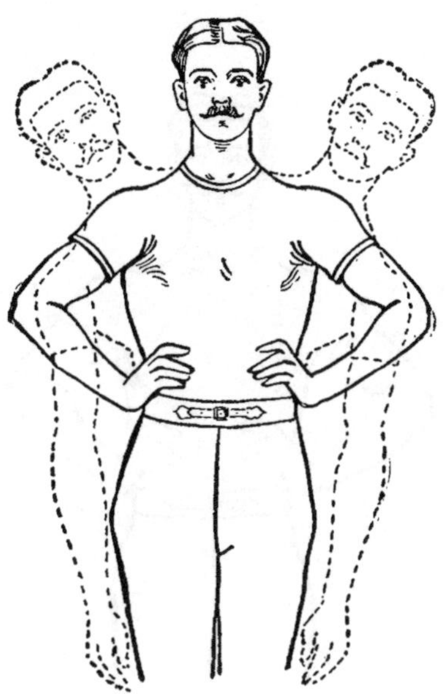

Bending—Waist Muscles

Twisting

Stand erect. Place the hands on the ribs. Weight of the body firmly on both feet. *Turn* as far to the *left* as possible *without moving the feet.* Keep the head in its relative position to the body; that is, when facing square to the front. By observing this caution the head will not turn in advance of the body.

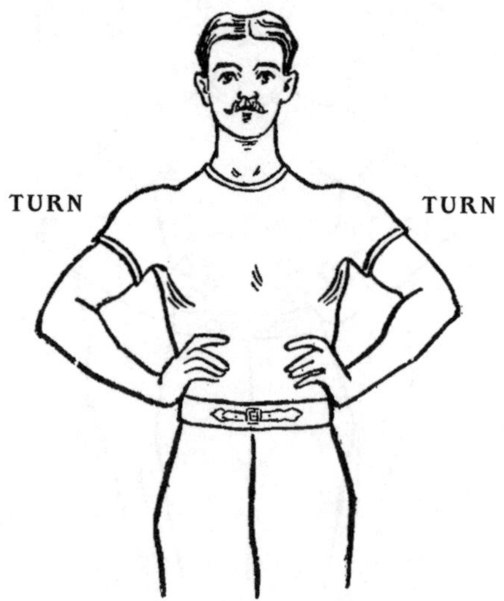

Twisting or "Liver Squeezer."

When turned as far as possible to the left, turn back slowly to position; then as far to the *right* as possible, keeping the feet solid upon the floor, not allowing them to turn when the body turns.

This exercise, especially the turning to the right, is known to thousands of my pupils as:

❦

The Liver Squeezer

This is the simplest, the most efficacious, the least expensive remedy for a torpid liver that was ever given to the public. Try it, also, when you have a bilious headache. Because you feel the least like exercising is no indication that exercise should not be taken.

Exercise, proper exercise, will rest you when ordinarily tired, if not too much exhausted. When one is tired it is seldom that he is tired *all over.* If this be true then one set of muscles has been overworked. Rest them by working some other set. When tired walking, run a little while. When the brain is tired work the body.

This matter of *resting* by changing the *mode* of work I saw exemplified by some workmen employed in a large foundry in Chicago. I had occasion to pass them every day during the noon hour. The noon meal had been eaten. Many of the workmen were *resting* themselves (after their laborious work of the morning) by playing ball, and that most vigorously.

Liver Squeezer—Turn; left; right (five times).

NOTE—For special or individual work, not less than ten times each way.

STATIONARY RUNNING

Running, or some form of exercise requiring deeper and fuller breathing than is obtained by walking, should be indulged in daily.

It is not convenient to practice running on the crowded thoroughfares of our large cities. We might be running for health and pleasure, and get just the opposite. The liability to arouse suspicion would also be a barrier to such a form of exercise. But we can obviate that difficulty by *stationary* running.

Incline the body forward as if starting to run a race. Close the hands and place them on the chest to keep it active and to keep the arms from swaying. Close the mouth and *keep it closed.* Run, but do not move out of the position in which you are standing. Begin slowly, increase the speed, then more slowly again at the finish. Stand in the open, moving air, if possible, if not, by an open window.

Running—Go; halt (fifty steps).

NOTE—Count (mentally) each step as the foot touches the floor. For special work, the running should be from 200 to 500 steps.

THAT TIRED FEELING IN THE SMALL OF THE BACK

Have you ever had it? Did you ever find any special exercise that would relieve it? Well, here is one.

Stand erect, the weight of the body equally divided over both feet. Place your hands on the hips. Make yourself as tall as possible from the chest, but do not lift the feet from the floor, even to the extent of slightly raising the heels. Reverse the natural order of the position of the feet; that is, instead of the heels together and the toes turned out, put the toes together and separate the heels. Slowly, first with the one foot then with the other, separate the heels as far apart as possible, keeping the toes of the shoes touching. Keep the body well up.

Small of the Back—Place hands; toes; tall; separate heels.

NOTE—*Once* should give instant relief.

❦

HOBBY HORSE

Every one rides a hobby. This is one that will greatly benefit you, the special object being *elasticity of the leg muscles*, thus causing one to be "light on the feet." It will also give you *better breath control* and *greater lung capacity, if* you keep the *mouth shut.* This should be done not only when exercising, but *after* the exercise until the breathing is normal.

The name is significant, as the exercise is suggestive of one riding a hobby-horse. The upper portion of the body, pivoted at the hips, moves backward and forward, while the legs, alternately, extend forward and backward.

Place the hands on the hips. Extend the right leg forward, sway the body backward. As the right leg comes back to position raise the left leg immediately and extend it backward, swaying the body forward. Alternately touch the right and left foot to the floor, touching only the *ball of the foot*, and, as nearly as possible, always touching the feet in the *same place.*

Hobby Horse—Place hands; ready; ride; rest (three times).

Note—Continue for a few seconds. For individual work, continue until the breathing is very deep and laboured.

❦

Stair-Climbing

I say stair *climbing,* because the majority of those who have stairs to ascend *do* climb, especially women.

There is no one exercise that is more healthful or more invigorating than going up and down stairs, provided that the air in the halls is pure.

The benefits are threefold: *strengthening the lung muscles, increasing the lung capacity* and giving *breath control.*

But, like everything else, there is a *right* and a *wrong* way. Wife and I have tested its virtues by walking up the steps of every monument in this country. (Washington Monument, 898 steps.)

When the public school teachers learn by experience the benefits derived from this mode of exercise, they will no longer "*dread those horrid stairs,*" but will consider them a blessing, a great boon to humanity. Furthermore, they will go earlier than usual to school in order to go up and down the stairs several times before the regular exercises of the day begin. Then, should they feel tired when the day's session is over—which they *should* not, and which they *would* not if they devoted ten minutes morning and afternoon to giving the pupils this series of exercises—they will, before going home, ascend and descend the stairs many times for the purpose of resting.

The Right Way

There are *three special points* to observe:

First—Touch *only the ball of the foot* to the step in passing either up or down. The planting of the whole foot upon the step and heavily striking the heel is in direct violation of the physiological principle concerning the jarring of the brain, the cerebellum.

Second—Incline the body forward, but *do not bend it at the waist.* Keep the chest active, and thus avoid stooping and interference with the breathing.

Third—*Keep the mouth shut.* (Very difficult, especially if two or more persons are together.) See that every inhalation is diaphragmatic, not clavicular.

Avoid talking when ascending, and *especially when reaching the top* of the stairs. Do not puff out the little breath that is left. *The mouth should not be opened* under any consideration *until the breathing is normal.* If the breathing is full and deep and laboured, there is all the more need of keeping the mouth closed until the heart and lungs have resumed their normal condition. By observing this last caution one will also be benefited *vocally* by the increase of volume and by resonance.

In descending the stairs the body should be erect. Bend only the knee joint, touch only the ball of the foot, descend lightly, gracefully, noiselessly, yet firmly.

Just a word in conclusion. In order to reap the richest harvest from the foregoing series, one must exercise *regularly* every day. Do it as a religious duty. Be as regular in your exercises as you are in your *devotions*—no; as regular as you *ought* to be.

When to Exercise

Never allow a morning of your life to pass without taking the bowing exercise *fifty* times. Take the joint exercises in the morning and the muscle exercises at night just before retiring. Always take the *special* exercises (such as rising on the toes, etc.) directly after any long-continued mental effort.

Midway between breakfast and the noon hour is the best time, physically considered, for any form of vigorous exercise.

Follow the morning and evening exercises with a sponge or hand bath of cold water, if you have sufficient vitality for reaction; if not, lukewarm water.

Do not allow yourself to get chilled when bathing. Put a handful of salt in the bowl of water; it will strengthen and invigorate you and prevent your catching cold—or the cold catching you.

Last, but not least of all, if you wish the body to be a fit temple for the indwelling of the soul, three things observe with care—*what* you *eat, what* you *drink, what* you *think.*